Miraculous Sickness

Miraculous Sickness

ky perraun

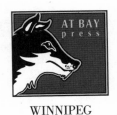

WINNIPEG

Library and Archives Canada cataloguing in publication is available upon request.

ISBN 978-1-988168-57-9

Printed and bound in Canada.

This book is printed on acid free paper that is 100% recycled ancient forest friendly
(100% post-consumer recycled).

With the generous support of the Manitoba Arts Council.

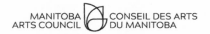

MANITOBA ARTS COUNCIL   CONSEIL DES ARTS DU MANITOBA

First Edition

10 9 8 7 6 5 4 3 2 1

atbaypress.com

ACKNOWLEDGEMENTS

The following poems have previously appeared in earlier versions:

"Appointment" – *Grey Matters*, 2003.

"Clinical Observation," "Tranquilized," "Miraculous Sickness," "Lotus Blossoms on the Pond of Eternity," (also won the Poetry on the Wards contest, 2009), "Shrinkipoo," (also placed third in the Brainstorm Poetry Contest, 2009), "Bedlam Beckons" – *Paging Dr. G*, Right Heart Press, 2010.

"No Cure" – *The Prairie Journal of Canadian Literature*, Issue 51.
"Side Effects" – *As One Cradles Pain*, David Fraser, editor, 2012.
"Silent Plague" – *In New Light*, Miriam Harrison, Dinah Laprairie and Ken Lillie-Paetz editors, 2013 (also received honourable mention in the Brainstorm Poetry Contest, 2009).

****

Details of the case of Jeffrey James at Toronto's CAMH ("Cracked," "Elegy for Jeffrey") were taken from Anthony Reinhart's article, "Avoid using restraints, coroner's jury urges," *The Globe and Mail*, October 11, 2008, updated March 13, 2009. Details of the case of James Proscope and the Mental Health Centre, Penetanguishene ("Cracked," "Hard Capsule to Swallow") were taken from Kirk Makin's article "Hospitals, judges at odds over how to handle mentally ill," *The Globe and Mail*, July 29, 2011, updated July

29, 2011; and Sean Fine's article, "Doctors tortured mental health patients, judge rules," *The Globe and Mail*, June 8, 2017.

The author wishes to thank The Canada Council for support during the creation of this work.

Greg Hickmore provided invaluable editorial advice on early versions of this manuscript.

I would like to thank my editors at At Bay Press, Kristian Enright, and Karen Clavelle, for their insightful, thoughtful and intelligent suggestions, comments and questions. Any shortcomings of this book are despite their input.

Finally, to all who have documented the plight and treatment of those with mental illness throughout the ages, from papyrus scrolls to documents online, a deep bow of gratitude. Without their efforts, the histories of that marginalized community (of which I am a part), would have been forgotten. In particular:

Madness in Civilization – A Cultural History of Insanity, Andrew Scull; *Great and Desperate Cures*, Elliot S. Valenstein; *In the Sleep Room: The Story of the CIA Brainwashing Experiments in Canada*, Anne Collins; *Surviving Schizophrenia: A Family Manual*, E. Fuller Torrey, MD; *The Invisible Plague: the rise of mental illness from 1750 to the present*, E. Fuller Torrey and Judy Miller; *The Faber Book of Madness*, Roy Porter, editor; *Medicating Schizophrenia – A History*, Sheldon Gelman; "History of Schizophrenia," from schizophrenia.com; Historical Roots of Schizophrenia," Martin L. Korn, MD;

"Historical Roots of Schizophrenia, History of Institutionalization/

Treatment," from Medscape.org; "Donald Ewen Cameron," from Wikipedia; "R.D. Laing; Summary of Important Concepts," http://web.sonoma/d/daniels/laingsuummary.html; "How It Was: Terror and Water-Boarding the Insane in Philadelphia," Dan Agin; "The First Asylums in Canada: A Response to Neglectful Community Care and Current Trends," Sam Sussman, PhD, *Canadian Journal of Psychiatry*, Vol. 43, April 1998; "The History of the Psychopharmacology of Schizophrenia," Heinz E. Lehmann, MD, Thomas A. Ban, MD; *Canadian Journal of Psychiatry*, Vol 42, March 1997; "Historical Synopsis – The Department of Psychiatry at the University of Toronto," from the U of T website; *The Globe and Mail*: October 11, 2008, updated March 13, 2009; July 29; June 8, 2017.

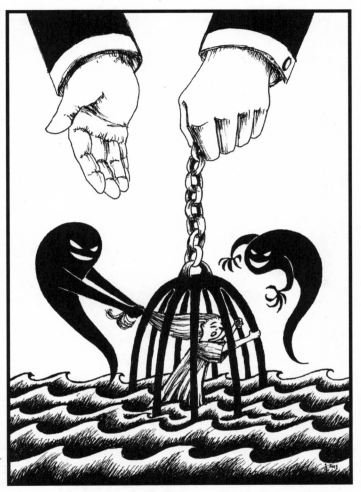

Agonies by the Conscious and Subconscious, Izabela Ciechanowska

For Vic, my soul mate, and R.K., my poetry mentor.

PEERS

"It took quite a bit to convince us that anything as pedestrian as biochemistry was relevant to something as profound and poetic as what I was going through. For me to admit the possibility that I might not have gone nuts again had they given my pills when I left was a tremendous concession.

"It's such a poetic affliction from inside and out, it's not hard to see how people have assumed that schizophrenia must have poetic causes and that any therapy would have to be poetic as well. A lot of my despair at ever getting well was based on the improbability of finding a poet good enough to deal with what happened to me."

– Mark Vonnegut, *The Eden Express*

POET ENOUGH

Two decades of pointing to the moon
of lunacy, and the finger is studied.
The fantastic, the surreal experience of madness
too complex, intricate, divorced from reality
to do justice with words. I am not poet enough,
though I am mad.

I was wont to lie on the couch of analysis,
to free associate and wax poetic, but was instead
offered pills, syringes, liquids chased by juice,
by science-oriented doctors wearing white coats.

When my mind was sufficiently righted by those
pedestrian means, I struggled to convey the land
I'd travelled, but could produce only blurred photos
in words, static representations of the dynamic dream.

Now I depict the care given those with similar afflictions,
in poems written from recovery, and pray I am poet
enough to give voice to those whose silence screams
to be acknowledged. Invisible victims, whose suffering
at the hands of healers was inexcusable. I speak for them now,
in verse, identify with their impotence in the face of authority,
their confusion at minds gone awry.

A poetic condition, as the future MD noted, one that goes
beyond mere fact, with a history of treatment that reads
like a horror novel, or a very dark poem.

SILENT PLAGUE

(for Colin)

Remembering those who have fallen
by their own hands, victims of misfiring
neurotransmitters, society's cruelty,
the great barnyard pecking order,
which leaves those of different persuasions
bleeding and scarred, the man toasts the ghosts
of comrades and neighbours in his tenth-floor cell.

The urgent traffic on the avenue
not quite erasing the pain of small-town streets,
the sounds of the city a backbeat
to the echoing taunts of the narrow-minded
and unenlightened citizens of isolated bergs everywhere.

The nightly news does not report the toll
of human anguish, providing denial required
to ensure a place in heaven for those
who found life too painful to endure.

The man locks his list of the departed,
to be taken out and read aloud in a future ritual,
his tribute to an act of despair and despondency
he understands all too well, and vows to fulfill
his duty on earth – to fight for the rights
of the disenfranchised,
to prevent the list from lengthening,
to survive and save others from suicide,
the silent plague of the sorrowful.

CECILIA MCCOUGH, STUDENT, ASTONOMER, ACTIVIST, WRITER

That high, fine intelligence, star catcher, voyager
of the heavens, laid low by visions of evil, the colours
red and white triggering terror. The torture of
ubiquitous hallucinations: horrible clowns, demonic,
peopling the audience as you testify about your affliction
in public, to be broadcast to the world.

A serious student, suffering from schizophrenia, you knew
there were others on campus whose minds betrayed them.
You formed a safe haven of camaraderie, healing, a support
group built on acceptance, empathy.

You discovered a star, despite your diagnosis. The heavens
will never be the same.

"I am not a monster," you assert, addressing the popular concept
of those who suffer from psychosis.

Watching you on the small screen, I am in awe
of your intellect and courage. Thank you for your courage
and honesty, your battle against stigma.

The heavens will never be the same.

HER MOTLEY FLOCK

The mad mingle freely. *Half of Geel is crazy,*
the other half-crazy, the saying goes.

Difficult to tell the boarders from the regular citizens.
Home. Sanctuary. Peace. Utopia for the ill, the small
Belgian city, site of St. Dymphna's shrine, the patron
saint of the mentally ill, grew as families left their afflicted
members with the peasant farmers, who welcomed
the extra hands.

The tradition continues, a model of community inclusion,
though numbers have declined drastically.

A home, a bed, a room. A family to return to, to shelter
the afflicted. Freedom from restraints, locked wards.
                    Meaningful occupation.   Acceptance.

Inclusion therapy, purpose and belonging. Visible,
part of the community, the daily rhythms of the city,
dancing to the melodies their minds compose,
resonating with harmonies of love, the saint at the centre,
smiling benevolently on the cobblestone and crosses,
the comings and goings of her motley flock.

THERESA

Theresa wields her walker like a weapon
as the bus rumbles to a stop. She nudges
passengers with her chrome implement, a queen
dispersing peasants from her path.

In thrift stores she circles shoppers whilst chanting
a spell, in rhythm with her wheels' rotations,
defying the silent clerk to intrude on magic.

In the streets she screams at passers-by,
accusing them of treason.

Only to her nurse does she speak softly,
as the syringe enters her arthritic hip.
The monthly medicine is a ritual
performed by scrub-suited angels
who, in the hierarchy of heaven, deserve respect,
which Theresa doles out like lint-furred pocket mints
on the pew of the examination table.

CRACKED

This solitary art, with the weight of millennia
bearing down on tight shoulders, this telling
of woe and epiphanies, this long look
at the history of suffering and treatment
renders me fragile as an egg, and as nascent.

In Canada, in the 21st century:
Jeffrey James, 34, dead after a week of restraints
James Proscope, held in filth for 61 days
in the Mental Health Centre, Penetanguishene.

Countless tortured across the world
throughout the history of mental health
treatment, in the name of care.

A small fissure appears on the surface of my shell.
I peer out, prepare to write my way clear of my confines,
to be set free by the Muse, and reveal the truth
of those whose minds betrayed them, as, often,
did those who were charged with their care.

HARD CAPSULE TO SWALLOW

On June 7, 2017, a judge ruled that doctors tortured
patients in the Oak Ridge, Penetanguishene facility
in central Ontario in the late 60s and 70s. A maximum
security institution, Oak Ridge housed the hard-to-handle.
The doctors conducted experiments with drugs,
solitary confinement, and brain washing. They chained
naked patients together in what they called
The Capsule Program, kept them in a continually-lit,
windowless room and fed them through straws.
Some were kept with ankles bound together and tied
to their wrists.

One of the doctors wrote that Nazi techniques
could be cited, were it not that the afflicted
did not choose their values, and that the medical team
should use "force, humiliation, and deprivation"
as they saw necessary to change the patients' values,
right their chemistry, and overcome their apparent internal confusion.

The judge quoted the Hippocratic Oath
before passing judgement.

MODERN DAY EULOGY

(Elegy for Jeffrey)

Palm. Pulse. Stroke. Reprieve.
Pleasure overriding pain. Commands
for the quickening stroke, out among
the angels and spies, by the fishbowl
of scrubs and thick files, where staff
congregate, hungry for silence.

Loud sounds demanding cessation. Desire
pulls. Release eclipses reason.

They converge and tackle, these loud-sound
makers. Sting of the syringe. The bed
slams into his face. Leather straps, taut,
on wrist, ankle. Oblivion.

An empty room ebbs in and out of focus.
Night becomes day five times over.
Ache in the limb, a tightness.

Release.

Then nothing. The patient is dead.
A clot converged on his lung, stealing
his breath. Gasp.

Black lives matter.
Jeffrey James, 34, patient at Toronto's CAMH.
RIP.

Whether by cop or doctor, the tragedies astound.

STATES OF SCHIZOPHRENIAS

You want to make it better
with your words, your pills,
your programs. You have us
perform parlor tricks for tokens,
grant us privileges of small freedoms
at the price of dignity.

Father/nurse, may I play Monopoly?
        The ward is Park Place, and
        I am a car.

Mother/doctor, may I take a walk?
        A long one, on a short pier?

Reduced to the status of ill-tempered toddlers,
force-fed mind-numbing drugs, shuffling,
slack-jawed to bland, finely-chopped meals.

You promise
You promise
You promise

But rarely deliver

Rights
Shelter
Pleasure

We are tagged and tranquilized,
then sent to the streets
of spike-crusted doorways
and enterprising hustlers.

Your ledgers are balanced
on our backs. You show
a good return, the playpens
you erect from the skeletons
of theories are cost-effective,
cheaper than asylum
in its most generous sense.

We wander off, disillusioned,
to be summarily captured
in a terrible dance of the damned.

Tra la la
do si do
and it's one for the fast track to Bedlam
the long, looping road home.

LOOKING BACK

LOOKING BACK

I cannot take myself
out of the equation, I realize
as I devour exposés of mistreatment.
"There but for the grace of ... [science] [compassion] ..."

I know what works, at least
what allows me to function, albeit
on the margins. I see it in my peers.
No metrazol shock, near drownings,
organ removal or beatings would do
the trick. No – it is these imperfect
medications that calm us
and set our minds right.

I am using an afflicted organ
to organize these facts. The crutch
of neuroleptics allows me to limp
through the reportage and glean
salient points from the invective.
I am hyper-aware of my vulnerability
as I peruse the studies of victims, of casualties.
This is a subjective treatment of an age-old issue.

My worry worn notes bear the watermarks
of experience.

BOOK OF HEARTS

An ancient Egyptian papyrus, probably extant from copies made of texts from 3400 BCE, in a chapter called "The Book of Hearts," describes madness, heart and mind considered synonymous. This was one of the earliest known mentions of mental illness, which was viewed as a combination of blocked channels
and the existence of angry gods and evil spirits.

In the land of the Pharaohs, the stricken.

In the shadows of the pyramids, the ill.

Madness always with us, from time immemorial.

SONOROUS REMEDY

Saul, after feasting on the Philistine's plenty,
was stricken with an evil spirit. Having disobeyed
the Lord, he now required music to exile the demon
inhabiting his soul.

Sweet harp song of David! Melodious exorcism –
notes wound round the vile intruder, banishing,
soothing madness.

Make a joyful noise! Calm the raging mind.
Songs medicinal, righting the afflicted.

Sonorous remedy.
Spirit cleansed by sounds evoked
from the instrument of angels, harmony
of heaven and man, each string tethered
to solidity, grounding the king to eternal truth,
his mind's muscle moored and obedient
to the will of the Father.

Let the choir sing "Amen."

NEBUCHADNEZZAR II

Invocation
"Great king of Babylon, second to none,
whose dream of the mighty tree signaled
seven years' exile in the land of the beast,
hair like eagle feathers, nails like claws,
devouring grass and all manner of beastly repast,
return to us, humble and with a mouthful of praise
for the Lord Thy God who maketh all whole."

That madness came in all hours of man,
is evidence of this so human affliction.

That Nebuchadnezzar II recovered is testament
to the resilience of the mind, or some would say,
the grace of the Lord.

Some recover with no treatment. Some would say
prayer is the cure.

I say lunacy is nothing new, and favours no one;
the moon reflects light on all manner of human
(oh-so-human) beings, regardless of power or station.

That some fall under its sway is evidence
of no earthly exemption.

ANCIENT HEALER

Christ cast demons into swine —
ancient healer, purifying mind.

The beasts ran off of a cliff
to the sea, healing the rift

between high, fine and holy
and the mundane, Christ solely

responsible for the miracle,
calming the hysterical

while villagers fed
the afflicted, it is said

showing great compassion
by sharing their rations

and the sane and satiated
the Good Lord created

lived harmoniously by the sea
madness curable, it seems.

GALEN IN ISLAM
(Galen of Pergamon, 129 AD – c. 200/c. 216)

The founder of psychotherapy, erudite and influential, held sway over the Islamic world. Discourse to treat mental disease, caused by "alterations in the equilibrium of the body."
No mind/body split here!

Flash forward: the first hospital constructed in the near East in the late 8th century. By the 12th century, medical facilities appear in all large Islamic towns, but Avicenna, father of early modern medicine, Islamic Golden Age's polymath, author of the Canon of Medicine, whose star shone brightly until the 18th century, deems beatings therapeutic. The afflicted are often chained, struck repeatedly.

Cuppings, purges, blood-letting. Humor-balancing diets, opium and oils, herbs and milk to the head, forerunners of today's pharmacopeia.

No: talk, talk, talk soothed the most savage! A privilege then, as it is today, to give voice to inner turmoil.

Woe to the patient. Woe. Galen, cherry-picked. Only chemicals, not words.

Flash forward: 15-minute consultations with a script the answer to all existential questions.

Woe to the patient. Woe.

OATH

(Hippocrates of Kos, c. 460—357 BCE)

Brain the seat of emotions, mental activity. Humors, those visceral liquids, determine temperament.
Too much blood: nightmares, terrors. Too much phlegm: mania. Melan (black) chole (bile): despondency.

In those ancient days before neuroleptics, psychotropics: purges, emetics, bleeding, changes to manner of living prescribed.

Father to physicians, his oath remains, though harm was later done in the treatment of the mad. Science backtracked, ill-advised. Drunk on power, Hippocrates' progeny committed all manner of crimes on unwitting patients. "Do no harm" paid lip service, his legacy tainted by questionable intent.

FULL CIRCLE

I.

Hippocrates, prescient physician, proto endocrinologist, ancient Greek seer of the psyche, European father of modern medicine, prophet of brain science, summoned Aesculapius, with his snake and staff, to render compassionate physicians in their pursuits of cure. "Do no harm" repeated to this day, humoral theory evident in the lexicon: *sanguine, phlegmatic.*

Do no harm, indeed. Our hero thought the womb the seat of all diseases of women, a sentiment that later led to unnecessary hysterectomies and the theory of hysteria. From the days before Christ to the era of Freud, women have been subjugated to cruel and unusual interventions. Sisters misunderstood by the scholars of healing, mutilated and repressed, robbed of organs and free speech.

II.

The 1990s – decade of the brain, neurotransmitters the new humours – too much dopamine = Parkinson's,
too little = schizophrenia; too little serotonin = despair, too much = toxicity. Full circle we dance around notions of healing and healer. Forsaken, the notion of schizophrenogenic mother, woman as culprit and cause. Still, sisters are cautious as deer caught in headlights

of cruel scrutiny, their arms crossed over abdomens, protecting what was once seen as their burden.

HOLY FOOL

Plato and Socrates had high praise for the alternative views of the mad – Bacchic, exotic, creative, prophetic, transformative – divine madness the way through to truth and mysticism.

The holy fool is a stock figure in literature throughout the ages, as though insanity conferred wisdom. The same sentiment can be seen in the works of the renegade psychiatrist R.D. Laing, with his accounts of 'breakthroughs.'

The high romance is not lost on us, we who carry the burden of delusions and hallucinations. It's like the masterpiece the million monkeys type – mine the ramblings for nuggets of profundity and one might find some – perhaps due more to momentary lucidity than flashes of brilliance shooting through the cracks in reason.

Sometimes we take refuge in our exalted status in the minds of a few who cling to the notion madness and genius are closely aligned.

Taken to heart, however, such esteem leads to grandiosity, and that is punishable by stigma.

ADMISSION TO BETHLEHEM HOSPITAL "BEDLAM" LONDON, c. early 18th c.

Sleight of hand, trickster, malicious,
big, fat, juicy lies, auto-concentric minds,
making of us beasts who devour the fields
or our own filth, who run on all fours.
Disappearing act of capital R reason for a season,
                    for all time.

Untamed, shackled, beaten. Naked, filthy
spectacle. The holiday crowd files by, gaping,
thinking, "There but for the grace of God ..."
and, "What creatures exist on God's green earth?"

In the common area, cacophony of mutterings,
floor defiled, bare feet pacing through the sewage.
Through barred windows the clean shining faces
of society peer – the alienists with scrutiny,
the orderlies with intent.

I dance on the edge of awareness
for the entertainment of my city.

I DO NOT WISH TO BE CALLED MRS.

Patrick Blair, in 1725, wrote of a married woman in his care,
who had abandoned her duties and spat "continually" while
sequestered in her room. He treated her with "frequent
bleedings, violent Emeticks, strong purgatives and potent
Sudorificks and Narcoticks" for a month before the water
cure. Three trials of being blasted with water from pipes
while seated on a chair in a tub took place before she
agreed to sleep with her husband and was declared cured.

"It appeared that in 90 minutes there was 15 Ton[s] of water
let fall upon her."

Some Observations on the Cure of Mad Persons
       – Patrick Blair

"I do not wish to be called Mrs.
I despise his name as I despise him –
his words, his mannerisms, his thrusting flesh
which brings me no joy, only distaste.
I stand firm in my convictions."

Later:
"I am weakened. When will this torture cease?
I am empty and frail. But I loathe the beast
they made me marry – his hairy hands and
flaccid gut are like a demon's – my flesh crawls
at the thought of lying next to him. Oh, let me
sleep forever!"

Still later:
"In order to save my life I go back to him.
I pretend I am glad. I will lie beneath him,
thinking of the seashore, shut my eyes
and endure his spasms. Oh, dear God,
that I might die!"

"The angels sing to me, but I dare not
harmonize. I am rocked in the bosom
of our savior and his disciples cover
me in swaddling. I am the mother of God,
me thinks, crucified nightly by that man
to better be with my heavenly hosts."

"I spit the taste of him from my tongue."

PUNISHMENT

Lin Shiyuan, in 1763 China, hurled a roof tile festooned with strips of paper bearing nonsensical words in the direction of Dingshang, the governor of Fujian.

What did his beleaguered brain mean to convey? What code would we need to crack? What delusions of persecution tortured him enough to strike out?

Executed for "Blithely circulating devious words, writing placards and rousing and confusing people's hearts," he was offered no asylum, only punishment, more than mere stigma.

I think of my own missives, sent out in desperation as the complex web of my delusions threatened to entrap me.

Grateful for my time and place of birth, I place a metaphorical stone on the grave of Lin Shiyuan.

CHINESE TEMPLE

Caged, incarcerated like a beast, inside the Chinese Temple, the patient, incoherent, terrified, was lowered into water, submerged, almost drowned, then raised to cling to life — and presumed sane. A dangerous practice, the inventor allowed (he who espoused humane treatments) but effective in calming the mind, or so it appeared as the patients lay supine sputtering, docile, reticent.

The smooth surface of the water a *tabula rasa*, the patient presumably erased of all evidence of madness.

CHINESE TEMPLE 2
(c. 1826)

They submerged witches to prove their guilt.
So, too, me, who has committed the crime
of insanity. But rather than conviction, submersion
is designed to cure my malady, I, who am already
incarcerated.

Locked in a cage, I am lowered into the pool.
At the point of death I am raised, sputtering,
gasping, lungs nearly burst.

Enervated, terrified, I am docile as a lamb.
I no longer pace and rave. I am an easy charge.
This the doctors take as proof of the efficacy
of their methods.

These men of medicine are demons incarnate. My flesh crawls.
Voices of hell still ring in my ears. I cower in corners.
I pray the staff will pass me by.

YOU WILL NEVER GIVE UP

Death is nothing, you say, you repeat
as the cage is lowered into the pool. Fools!
They think they can shock you into believing
what you see is not real. But you have seen the demons' work,
those shape-shifting faces, the expansion and contraction
of the flesh of your enemies. They swell and subside.
You recoil, gasp, sputter, emerge. Now you are spent,
but keep your thoughts and words to yourself.
You will never give up your mind, your truth, your power.

KING'S RATIONS

Even kings knew restraints. George III in a straitjacket, beaten,
chained into subjection. Starved and berated by his subjects in the
asylum at Lincolnshire, the monarch suffered all manner of horrors
and humiliation.

Your Highness! Give us a grin.
The kiss of the whip incites vocalizations
far removed from a speech. Mind your wrists,
shackled as they are. You slobber and slaver
for a spoonful of gruel. But you'll have none
today, Your Highness. Not until the madness
leaves. Not until you are sane.

God save the king from the "cure,"
as dreadful as the affliction!

Note: When the king's illness went into remission, Francis Willis,
who oversaw the asylum, was rewarded with a substantial pension.

THE TRANQUILIZER

c. early 19th century

They strapped my arms and legs to their crude, cruel chair, then secured a box over my eyes, blinding me. Still, the phantoms convulsed and repulsed, and the voices commanded, unabated.

Cold water applied to my head, warm water to my feet, designed no doubt to draw demons from my skull, only irritated and heightened the horror.

I hold still, bite my tongue, scream silently to appear dumb, until they release me, pleased with my docility.

I stay still and hushed. They are pleased. I am coddled, dressed and trundled off to bed.

The Tranquilizer is a delight to my keepers, a cure for my ills.

Only I know the voices continue.

SWINGING CHAIR

c. early 19th century

Swung like a ball tethered to a string, swung in circles by the attendant's crank of the handle; roped in and upright, swung till the stomach revolts and spasms ensue.

Swung, one's sense of what is human, lost. Stomach, bowels and bladder empty in quick succession.

Spun and slung till heaving, trembling, hairs on end and spasms rocking.

The alienist gloats – a cure! For, silenced and incapable, the patient does not stir.

Docile and manageable, the ward no longer troubles, praise the Lord! So, a reasonable sanity can be inferred.

OLD JONES AND THE SPREAD EAGLE CURE

(c. 1860s)

Demons wrestled into submission with whiskey and curses,
a long night made longer by time's thick consistency
in the beleaguered mind. Old Jones wandered in the street
in the general vicinity of his pauper's lodgings, arms flailing,
spittle shooting through grimacing lips, dressed in clothes
that had seen better days, beard long and wispy, breakfast crumbs
wagging in the strands as he cursed.

Notified by some good townsfolk, a beat cop escorted Old Jones
to the madhouse.

The next day orderlies tied Old Jones down, spread eagle, leather
across his chest and around his wrists and ankles, then dumped
water on his head while standing on a chair.

He nearly drowned.

Brought to the brink of death, Old Jones was quiet at last. A cure!

The orderlies half-carried Old Jones back to his cell. A report
of success was made to the superintendent. At last! The deaths
suffered in the wake of such treatment paled in comparison
to the new docility of the once troublesome Old Jones.

The superintendent took up his pen and with enthusiasm added
Old Jones' case to his speech he would give in a fortnight, guaran-
teed to draw the wealthy's afflicted relatives to his establishment.

The institute flourished, with good citizens flocking to its doors with difficult relatives in tow, hopeful of placing their burdens with the esteemed superintendent and his staff.

Old Jones remained in the madhouse, mute and terrified, requiring only the odd treatment to render him docile and mute.

Poster child of submission, Old Jones passed his days in his cell, little trouble at all, "cured" of his former enthusiasms by water from on high; the righting rains of medicine, a miracle.

CRUEL CUTS

I.

In the not-too-distant past, in the time before Steinem and Greere, before the ERA and suffragettes, a select group of doctors saw fit to circumcise women, to cure them of their ills.

Baby machines without sensual pleasure, they went on to mother-hood and docile domesticity, cured, the doctors declared, of their errant lusts.

II.

In a private clinic in Victorian England, women were deprived of their pleasure centers, that little organ of great grace, by a doctor who thought masturbation the cause of insanity, which could result in women wanting to work outside of the home.

If they didn't consent to clitorodectony, he said, they would go stark raving mad. For seven years Dr. Isaac Baker Brown, member of the Obstetrical Society of London, razed the sex of unwitting women, whose only crime was the desire for autonomy.

Eventually expelled from the Society, Brown was forced to cease his ministrations, but not until others also took up the knife, rendering independently-minded women pleasureless.

Docile mothers, dutiful wives, no longer seeking divorce, no longer craving emancipation, never to know the ecstasy of the intact female body again, all subjugated by the knife and the cruel cuts of misogyny.

FOCAL INFECTION THEORY

Teeth, tonsils, cervix, ovaries, colon – removed from patients exhibiting psychosis – focal infection theory.

Dr. Henry Cotton, operating in the 1920s, claimed such surgeries saved the state over $300,000 and had an 80 per cent success rate.

Excised, hollowed out, lighter in weight by the volume of flesh confiscated, but heavy with sedation, the patients-as-experiment deemed cured by virtue of new reticence, compliance, were paraded before an audience of eager medical men.

Cotton said the patients were infected, and, with no proof, removed pieces of their bodies, in the hopes of bolstering their minds. Dr. Cotton, hand-picking patients, had his moment of glory while those reduced by his treatment suffered their losses, learned to live, flesh lessened by the knife.

FULL FRONTAL

I.

"I'd rather have a bottle in front of me than a frontal lobotomy"
      – Tom Waits.

Holes drilled in skull, alcohol syringed into the cavities. Later, butter knife-like implements, and later still, entry through the nose and eye sockets. Treatment continued until the patient exhibited disorientation.

After: docility, incontinence, sometimes death.

By 1953, in the United States alone, over 200,000 lobotomies were performed, at times in hotel rooms. Flashing instruments and authority, mind meddlers professed to cure by destroying brain tissue blindly.

The unfortunate victims of medical science that survived drooled quietly in ward chairs while the staff, relieved of the necessity to control the agitated, praised the inventor, Egas Moriz, Nobel Laureate, 1949.

When psychotropic drugs proved effective, the lobotomy went out of fashion, though psychosurgery
may still be used in treatment-resistant patients today.

II.

Destroy what causes grief. Like generals on the battle ground, determined doctors waged war on the diseased brain by excision. The results were so striking, word spread round the world, and soon many were subject to the pick or spatula, rendered subservient, docile, with flattened emotions. Success! to the medical crew.

Demons excised, sucked clean from the brain cave. Disruptive patients rendered meek, hospital crews' dream. Around the world doctors drilled holes in beleaguered skulls. Or, for the less agitated, a pick was inserted in the nostril or eye socket. Swish, swish. Is the patient disoriented? We hit the mother lode —

She'll be no trouble at all
If she lives.

EFFICACY

There were success stories – the violinist resuming her career after lobotomy, having been rendered silent by madness, the doctor who took up his practice again after the surgery.

This kept the industry going, those blessed few who regained function in their former roles.

For the most part, patients were debilitated to mere shadows of their former selves, but docile enough the be easily handled. Some died.

Today psychosurgery is rarely performed, though it is more economical than additional asylum staff, which was the argument for its popularity.

FOOL

Plato and Socrates, before the common era, spoke of divine madness – prophetic, transformational, Bacchic, erotic, creative. One wonders if the schizophrenic were revered, honoured as R.D. Laing in the 20th century espouses

Oracle at Delphi, cave of vapours where the priestess, transported out of the quotidian realm of logic, writhed and prophesied. Essex House, London residence of the diagnosed, who danced and waxed poetic, with no fear of reprisal. Some solace there, despite recent findings that all is chemical, with no room for the interpretation of visions.

The Divided Self — A prophet with a fool entwined, Laing speaks of breakthroughs, reminiscent of the ancient Greeks.

Shamanic belonging, wounded healers holding forth on things mysterious.

Some solace there, though the 21st century is all elixir and alchemy, with little room for seers on the wards.

Prophets of old are today's patients, some scholars assert – *Muses, Madmen and Prophets*, the tome by Daniel B. Smith.

Some solace there, as we move through our days at the slow speed of life, with the future unknown and our reputations mundane, disregarded as "mad".

Our ravings dismissed, we sing in solitude, those days of holding court with the Gods mere footnotes, our fate to sit on the sidelines, former glory dim, the Holy Fool mere fool in this era of molecules.

SOUL DOCTORS

Mad doctors – all-too-sane physicians treating the frothing at the mouth, those flailing, loud blights on society.

Mad doctors – angry physicians whipping recalcitrant brains into shape with all manner of lashes, chains and devices, until moral treatment came into vogue, and asylums were constructed on vast, manicured lawns by reformers, Quakers among them, kindness and honest work prescribed.

Then they were known as alienists, as though studying life from other galaxies (which, I'm sure, their fate seemed at times, when confronted by illogic.)

In the early 20th century these fine fellows took on the rubric psychiatrists, from the Greek *psyche* (soul) and *techne latrike* (medical treatment).

Soul doctors. Repairing/re-evoking the spirit.

Holy host of narcoleptic.
Confessional of the office.
And the high, fine balm
of the good glances of the observer,
forever altering the observed.

FIELD OF NIGHTMARES

"Build it, and they will come," they say in *Field of Dreams*. Not only baseball fields, but asylums, filling to overcrowding as the mad multiplied in cities, ever-increasing numbers of lunatics (o, howl at the moon), striking fear in the hearts of citizens.

Some blamed train travel, some urban life. Some noted the Irish were overly represented in madhouses, some said alcohol. Some claim it was a plague, incidents of insanity on the rise since the 18th century, then levelling off in the 1950s.

Now the consensus has it, 1% of the population has schizophrenia – one in a hundred.

Some blame genes, some viruses. Mothers have been let off of the hook, schizophrenogenic has become an anachronism.

Nobody knows for certain. Only the suffering is indisputable.

SOLE EVIDENCE

A young Ewen Cameron arrived at the Brandon Hospital for Mental Diseases in 1929, full of vigour and ambition.

Inspired by the fever treatment of syphilis, he attempted to raise the bodily temperature of people with schizophrenia, placing them in an electric cage, but their pulses raced.

He read that red light promoted fertility in lab rats and plants, and so tried this on those with schizophrenia. He rigged up a cage and filtered light that resembled the transmission spectrum of blood. His patients lay naked in the light eight hours a day for as long as eight months.

He reported a degree of success worthy of recommendation, failing to note that those discharged were not chronic, his sole evidence his own observations.

THE HILL

They called it "The Hill," a place to threaten with, insult, disparage. For the young ambitious doctor Ewen Cameron, it was a large laboratory, a place to make his mark. Focusing on those patients for whom nothing seemed to work, he experimented with intense heat, and filtered red light.

When the patients' pulses soared in the electric cage, as their body temperature rose, he abandoned the fever cure for schizophrenia, and turned instead to red light filtered to resemble blood.

Up to eight hours per day for eight months, patients lay naked in a cage, in an effort to balance their endocrine systems.

When some were discharged, those who'd been hospitalized for the shortest term, Cameron wrote an article claiming victory. That the chronic patients were not improved he didn't bother to mention.

With no further proof than his own observations, he claimed success, though of limited potency.

The rule of thirds – one third of persons with schizophrenia improve with no treatment – held true. But ambition claimed the limelight and Cameron blew his own horn loudly.

What the patients endured did not seem to matter.

Hallucinating, locked in cages, subjected to inhumane treatment like so many lab rats, sweltering and stuck in blood-like light as the young maverick drooled over potential glory, the nightmare of madness, the cruel strivings of uncompassionate science.

Time would shine the light of horror on Cameron's ill-founded treatments, but not before so many victims had been harmed.

The legacy of "The Hill" is a chapter of shame in the annals of Canada's mental health system.

CONQUISTADOR

Ewen Cameron, preparing to give a paper on his psychic driving and depatterning efforts, chose his ten best cases to prove his methods, ignoring those that saw no improvement. As long as one-third of psychiatric patients improved, regardless of treatment, he would always have something to report.

Told he was skewing the results, he retorted that it was the way he did research. He saw his own mind as a better indicator of efficacy than any battery of tests. His psychologist on staff resigned in protest, after which Cameron criticized psychological testing.

Hubris, some charged. Others rallied behind Cameron, the visionary conqueror of the scourge of insanity. Cameron's bad science, for the most part, went unchallenged. He was seen as a conquistador, charging headlong into the land of madness.

REGRESS

Bosomy nurses, chosen for their matronly mammaries, coddled the afflicted, held their heads in their own shadowed laps, while distinguished doctors played daddy, stern yet loving, appearing sporadically, as good daddies did.

Undoing years of bad parenting, with its conflicting messages having sent offspring into the netherworld of psychosis, the medical staff played house, coddling and nurturing in the hope of righting their patients' minds.

In sleep- rooms and avant-garde residences, clients were swaddled and changed, babbled to in baby talk, re-raised to be sane. And yet, this did not cure. Years traversed in weeks, regress to pacifiers and bottles, the born-again inevitably reverted to old behaviours.

Thumb-sucking and mewing were interspersed with word salads. The days of free love were filled with hope of a solution to the problem of schizophrenia, with no side effects save the odd soiled diaper.

TABULA RASA

Ewen Cameron, august head of the World, the Canadian, and the
American Psychiatric Associations, and the Allen Memorial Insti-
tute in Montreal during the 1950s and early 1960s, wanted the
Nobel Prize so badly he could tolerate no opposition. Supported
in part by the CIA, through agencies formed to fund brainwash-
ing experiments, Cameron labored to find a cure for madness,
which could secure him the prize. He sought to wipe the minds
of patients clean, then write new scripts on the blank slates of
their psyches. This he did through "depatterning" and "psychic
driving" – repeated shock therapies at up to 30 times the usual
dosages, drug-induced sleep that lasted weeks or months, and non-
stop broadcasting of taped messages, as well as the administration
of LSD to the unwitting sufferers.

Eventually, he abandoned his project, but left in his wake amnesi-
acs and shells of former patients.

Tabula rasa – that's what you aimed for,
pure, pristine blankness, stripped of concepts,
clean of madness. A naked slate you could
inscribe sanity on. A prize-winning project,
and you, Nobel Laureate, basking in the light
of your own science, which is intuition, no need
for proofs beyond your own hunches.

Tabula rasa – smiling infant-like, uncomprehending,
incontinent, babes to the world,
victims of massive doses of electricity
to the skull. Thirty times the usual dosage.

Depatterning, you called it. Not one to coddle,
you left humanity to your underlings.
Let them do the drudgery. Buxom nurses,
carefully chosen, mothered the patients.
Heads on laps, spoon fed.

Tabula rasa – to be filled with words,
phrases repeated endlessly for hours on end
through speakers in the room, propaganda supreme.
This the foundation for the new personality.
Psychic driving, you called it, with you at the wheel.

Tabula rasa – months long drug-induced sleep
rendered the charges docile, malleable.
Comatose, the sleepers needed to be turned, fed,
toileted. This the nurses did, priding themselves
on unbroken flesh, lack of bedsores. Sleep therapy,
a name so innocuous, conjuring contented dreams
and soft pillows.

Tabula rasa – never the same, the patients
lost decades of memories, careers, life as they knew it.

And Cameron left, unscathed, to pursue his ambition elsewhere.

THORAZINE

Thorazine, an antihistamine, was later used as a calmative in surgery. Patients once mad became lucid under its spell, and the world of psychiatry changed.

Marketed as a treatment for nervous tension, vomiting, and all manner of ills, chlorpromazine gained popularity. Remarkable its effect on schizophrenia. The magic bullet, aimed at delusion, hallucination.

The emptying of the wards, the mass exodus of those formerly relegated to the back wards. Psychopharmacology the new gold standard. Better living through chemistry, the era of the brain rung in by that elixir.

New formulae, recipes tweaked continuously by long-labouring, lab-coated mavericks, followed on the heels of Thorazine. Hospital beds were reserved for acute cases, suicide attempts, and the premedicated. The schizophrenogenic mother a footnote in history, lobotomy and psychoanalysis gone the way of passing fancies.

Community treatment replaced extended incarceration. Though that model failed on many fronts, psychotropics proved a breakthrough. How they worked, however, remained a great mystery.

The serendipitous discovery, Thorazine, a benchmark. The great mystery of alchemy. The wonder drugs of neuroleptics, awaiting explanation.

IN THE ERA
OF RECOVERY

NO CURE

They tell me this medication could be deadly,
though deaths are rare, and summon my signature
on a form of consent. I comply, feeling brave
as a parachute jumper, desperate as a child starving
for a morsel of food. Life as it is, full of fear and torment,
risked for the sake of my mind's peace.

Weeks of hospital meals and the bloodthirsty syringe.
I make a fist for the tourniquet, tiptoe
past my depressed Christian roommate
when sleep eludes me
and the hollow-gut craving for nicotine
comes in the night of locked doors and curfews.

On the weekends, I cart a paper bag of cellophane envelopes
full of pills home, under the watchful eye of my lover.
I return to the ward Sunday at 9 p.m. sharp,
dodging the delusional as I stride
down the antiseptic hallway to the nurses' station,
with its sign-in sheet and thick files,
its permission slips, and locked drawers.

A visiting doctor waxes poetic
on the long-term benefits of the drug.
Another notes I am growing anemic.
Sedated, I watch the faces file past
my crib-like bed, feeling infantile and coddled.
            I am released.

Within a few days I am in a daze, dreams
and reality bleeding into each other
like a garish watercolour. I walk backwards
and babble on about nothing. I do not eat nor bathe.

I crawl to the mind-doctor. I am a vision of death.
He hands me a new prescription, and my name
is added to the waiting list for a hard-won bed.

I do not die, but taste the next world,
bitter as bile on my cracked, swollen tongue.
Pulled back from the precipice, I turn
to a book of Rumi and my own furrowed heart,
grateful for the latest chemical
and my days on the planet, now lucid.

These pills are a crap shoot. I cut my losses —
the empty calendar page, the pounds of flesh,
the vacant lecture hall seat. I cry out
my gratitude for a face undistorted
by the rolling tongue of side effects
and renew my vows of verse.

Cursed and blessed, I accept
the risks involved in living
with a disease of the mind. I clutch the hand
that is offered me, though no cure comes.

LOTUS BLOSSOMS ON THE POND OF ETERNITY

The drugs they doled out to tubercular patients
were the forerunners of today's antidepressants,
causing the patients' eyes to shine preternaturally bright,
their spirits to soar.

On the heights of Magic Mountain, the invalids
glow with beneficence, serotonin flowing
like clear waterfalls.

Today we dissect the literature like those unfortunate
formaldehyde-marinated frogs,
pins and placards naming turns of phrase,
while our brains, uncharted, vibrate,
gelatinous seats of the soul.

I would like to tell you how it is
inside this bony chalice, brain brimming
with barbituates and receptor-taming tonics,

But you would only measure my metre,
scan my lines for music, the mineral rights
of this landscape left to the mind doctors
and their laboratory lingo, so prosaic.

I move through your disciplined rooms,
foot-heavy and thick, subject, not author
of my fate, clutching my prescription
like a memo from G-d
my poems like formulae from forensics.

The neurologist scribbles haiku
on the wet windowsill. His tears of impotence
fog his lenses. Genuflecting before
the vast library of the mausoleum
he counts syllables like brainwaves
before locking his office against the erasure of night

Only to dream of receptors,
lotus blossoms on the ponds
of eternity.

TRANQUILIZED

When psychotic, I gathered experience like plucking raspberries
from the thorned bush of madness. Now, career patient,
I list my prescriptions like memorized verse, worship
at the monuments of the great minds of medicine
who in the not-so-distant past would charge a fee
to see me chained and foaming at the mouth.

Now, treated with the latest chemicals,
to lift my arm, I must dislodge boulders from the air,
each step a displacement of heavily-salted water,
each thought a chiseling in stone. The bed beckons.
In dreams, I can fly without effort.

Like a lioness sedated, I curl into the long grasses
of the morning, eyes heavy and harmless. The lamb
of literature lies down, unconquered.

GOOD WORLD

All of those years, raking fingernails across the faces
of saints, heart bristly as barbed wire, tearing the love
from your skull, my lover. All of those years I lashed
out from my wounding pain, concerned only
with the surface of things, having abandoned
all notions of subliminal beauty, when others knew
I was not right but I myself felt perfect and sane.

Now, late in the day I find my compassion
outside of my small self, and live to regret
those turbulent days of misfiring chemicals, those cold,
arid days of self-righteousness, when all
I could do was keep my own hand from firing
a gun at my skull.

I come to you now on the cloud of chemical salvation,
looking at Jesus from a new perspective, remembering
the existential wisdom of Buddha and Lao Tse
(consider the lilies, stay out of your own way),
and all manner of kindness bequeathed me
by you and at times, perfect strangers.
I come to you now, head bowed,
love coursing through my veins by virtue
of the nurse's syringe, and say

A lucid world is a good world.

SUBTYPES

Scientists love clean, neat categories. To label is to master, to name, to fathom. Thus, this disease, schizophrenia — paranoid, hebephrenic, catatonic, and simple.

The paranoid feels persecuted, and is at times grandiose.

The hebephrenic, or the disorganized lack coherence, have inappropriate expressions, or no expressions at all.

The catatonic: have behavioural disturbances — rigidity, posturing, stupor and mutism.

The simple: are plagued by apathy and withdrawal, flattened emotions, but experience no delusions nor hallucinations.

These categories failed to capture the experience of individuals, and so were abandoned. Some now speak of a spectrum. The lines are blurred, the manifestations of the illness infinite.

Now, it is common to speak of deficit and nondeficit schizophrenia, deficit being the prevalence of negative symptoms, and non-deficit largely treatment resistant.

Now, treatment is tailored to the individual, each one unique, categories less important than direct observation.

TIME, GENTLEMEN

"What seest thou else in the dark backward and abysm of time?"
    – Shakespeare

I.

"I have a problem with linear time," I declared back in the day, when I arrived late for a much-suggested appointment in the psychiatry department. My manic smile like a gill, the aquarium-like workspace of secretaries undulating in the heat of my psychosis.

I was handed a questionnaire, directed to the semi-circle of inhumane chairs by the automatic door that opened and shut soundlessly, a burlesque dancer's fan.

II.

The ink blots are clouds, dear doctor, and the sky is full of fighter jets headed somewhere. Laundry is to scholarship as sanity is to enlightenment. A rolling stone is naked, and people in glass houses let their arms hang limp.

Welts on my wrist where the watch's metal clasp touched flesh – like suicide scars. I am allergic to time. Dirty dancing of drugs in my brain, visions of van Gogh, stars melting across the macadam sky as I lie, parched, on the rubber-wrapped raft of the single bed.

III.

I arrive, on time, for the sting of the syringe, the thick syrup of lucidity, hands tied by chemistry and circumstance, small windows of wakefulness. I wait with others in the dense fog of neuroleptics. We are rarely seen punctually.

Time is a moving image of eternity, a wise man once said. I wait out my forever heavy-lidded and treading quicksand. Man-made construct, chafing this woman's spirit.

THE COLDEST MOMENTS

The coldest moment in the history
of your existence – heart, brain and bone
marrow freeze at the sentence you've been handed –
the word like an iceberg, crashing into your liquid
self-concept and up against your splintering spirit –
                              schizophrenia.

Later, on the slippery foam mattress
of a whitewashed rooming house cell,
you'll silently scream for cleansing tears,
the holy roil of an alarm clock to wake you
from the nightmare.

The deadening meds on the scarred nightstand,
the salvaged hospital bracelet, the treks
through sodden, foreign streets to the clinic
where the psychiatrist assesses your wooden
movements and mumbled responses, the library,
with its small selection of titles on the dreaded disease,
the cross-county phone calls, begging for reprieve.

"The thought of suicide has gotten us through
many a bad night," Nietzsche said.

Which you recite like a mantra,
until you, worn, forsake the prospect
of another round and swallow the whole
damned lot of your prescriptions
with a tequila chaser, salt burning your slack lips.

They force the liquid charcoal down your throat,
the syringe in your hip an enemy's arrow,
propelling you back into hell. Tossed back
into the land of the living, you vow to overcome
self-stigma, and recover, if nothing else, your dignity.

"A PLACE FOR THE GENUINE"

– Marianne Moore, "Poetry"

Discovered, mid-contempt for academia – the edifying nature
of verse. Apt observation for the attempted suicide,
words writ large against the pale, sterile backdrop
of a hospital room, with its three white carnations,
and lab coats padding by with mood scales and other
absurd questions.

What is significant is not the parking lot below
the unbreakable fifth floor window, nor the snores
of the benzo-dull roommate, nor the bland meals
arriving like clockwork and taken in bed, in the fashion
of the truly infirm. What is genuine may be entombed
in the phalanx of texts erected at the foot of the bed,
shielding the patient from the prying eyes of the mop-
wielding janitor, and informing all visitors that truly
noble thoughts reside behind the glassy eyes and
blank face, but only a sober archeologist could unearth
them.

"… the same may be said for all of us, that we
do not admire what/we cannot understand,"
Moore asserts, but I dare disagree – lines swimming
in a drugged fog mystify, cry out for decoding, contrast
the clinical charts and medication encyclopedias, compel
one to be admitted to the ranks of the truly articulate,
an ambition borne of desperation, which is as close to
admiration as one can come with a belly full of charcoal
and a plastic hospital bracelet identifying one as the charge
of a psychiatrist.

This poem I understood, and, hungry for the genuine, took
solace in its staggered lines and foot-noted quotes. Perhaps
there was hope, authenticity, beyond the petty details
of my disappointment, my truncated existence.

MIRACULOUS SICKNESS

"What about all the psychotics
in the world?
Why do they keep eating?
Why do they keep making plans
and meeting people at the appointed time?
Don't they know there is nothing,
a void, an eyeless socket,
a grave with the corpse stolen?
Don't they know that God gave them
their miraculous sickness
like a shield, like armour
and if their eyes are in the wrong
part of their heads, they shouldn't complain?
What are they doing seeing their doctors
when the world's up for grabs."

Letters to Dr. Y., January 12, 1969
      – Anne Sexton, "Poetry"

Medication, that oily brain balm,
greases thoughts, which slip
'round circumstance, wriggle and writhe
across document and prayer rug.

I've no delusion my sickness protects me –
it kills, and requires the taming power
of chemistry, therapy, schedules and plans.

My sickness is not miraculous. I go about
my business or die, simple as that.
These sidewalks do not reject my shuffling feet.
The buses do not abort me. The clocks are synchronized
and I obey, grateful for the predictable rhythm.

And you, belletrist, raped in the mouth
by a turgid exhaust pipe, let them win,
the naysayers and ticker tape crowd,
the romantic undergraduates idealizing madness.

Your small books.
Your brief life.

KING OF THE WARD

You enter, king of the ward, in your white lab coat
and sensible shoes, observe and record, report
of our activity measured and weighed against the charts
of high culture. You listen with an ear tuned
to a taut string you pluck while the orchestra sits,
instruments poised for the injection, the restraints.

We do not underestimate the power given you
by the state. We demure and bend to your will,
freedom a privilege you dole out like candy. Larger
than life, you preside over your flock, herd us into small
cells which reek of chemicals and despair.

We cannot tell you how the light in the asylum burns,
only show you the wounds, beg for a salve.

MAJOR TRANQUILIZERS

More brace than straitjacket, the chemicals steady
the mind. More brake than accelerator, the going
is slow. More eraser than chalk, the slate dusty
but blank. Grandiosity gone. Phantoms dissolved.
Voices silenced.

Vision blurred, belly backed up, muscles stiff, tongue
stuck to the roof of the mouth. Unquenchable hunger.
Systemic stuttering, accumulation of fat.

Through fog and quicksand, dusk and dim, the medicated
shuffle, harmless and dull. When the back wards emptied,
they emerged, drool and writhing tongues, a grimace and
eye whites. Now they rent rooms and congregate in NGOs,
smear paint and crochet placemats, though some enter
society a-blazing, making prognoses lies, shouting out
about stigma, restraints, paternalism, tremors of lithium
and passion, squared shoulders of dystonia and resolve.

Brain balm, dirty as a blue-collar joke, greasing square pegs
right into pigeonholes, or, miraculously, up to the heavens,
where even angels let them slip from their clutches.

ABILIFY

Subtle, this pill, my poems no longer
laundry lists of despair, my smile fluid,
the starch washed from my face.
I swallow happiness each day with breakfast.

Alchemical bliss, the brain unfettered, that
octopus slain that once choked my mind.
Metaphors flow from the pulse of grey matter,
the left prefrontal cortex plump with blood.
O, happy day.

The path I've travelled is flecked with semi-
precious stones, not the land mines of recent
ruminations. Casual words caught for eternity
no longer ring with malice. The humans who raised
me had all good intentions, their scarred psyches
conspiring to shield me from a similar fate. And if
their ministrations at times lacked delicacy, it was
through no fault of their own, just as my clumsy
erratic behaviour was the product of ignorance, affliction.
All is forgiven in the wake of this tiny oval tablet
and the examined life it allows. Hallelujah!
O holy host of high science, O philosopher's stone
melting like ice on the heat of my tongue!

REVOLVING DOORS

The mental health system is a labyrinth, with many false doors, dead ends, right angles, blind spots and trick questions asked at every turn.

Who, in your delusion, do you think you are? There is a pill to cut you down to size, aimed right at your sex Soon, that will go numb, and you won't be inclined to mate. And your arms – those must be restrained by these handy leather bracelets. See how they match the drab hospital gown?

The gurney is a fine slab, reminiscent of the morgue. Soon, you will die to yourself, and we shall build you up, notion by notion, till you comply like a child with our many rules and regulations.

You'll jump through hoops, make nice and be quiet. We can't have you in better neighborhoods, so it's off to the ghetto with you. Trust us, you'll adapt. If you wander into shopping districts, there'll be spikes on the ledges you may be tempted to rest upon.

Take two of these with water at five a.m., then one of those with lunch, and these three at bedtime. Don't get them confused!

Fill out these forms to get a refill. (In triplicate please, notarized and stamped.)

If you lose your ID, it's off to jail with you, so be careful.

Try to stay awake. The bus driver is not a babysitter. Wipe the drool from your chin. Look smart!

(Repeat unto death.)

IN THE ASYLUM

Mirages and drought, lighting in the left hip
where medicine enters.

The guard, home-grown and handsome,
sits perched on a bright metal chair.

Thin cot juts from the seclusion room wall –
small comfort. Clenched-muscle musings.
Cigarettes on the hour.

Small cups of sanity, incandescent beauty
in brick rooms of the nay-saying, isolated mad.

Billboard teeth of motivational speakers.
Congealed gel of craft room paint.

We mark minutes with lengths of ash,
the intervals between screams,
our selves lost in long hallways.

DEMENTIA PRAECOX

Aphasia. Alogia. Anhedonia. Anosognosia.
Symptoms like sisters in a thick Russian novel,
set in Siberia. You shiver.

Your doctor puts on a brave face, but his gaze
tears from yours and returns to the file.

The brain racing full speed into the twilight of reason.
No cure, only containment.

Mirror, mirror, on the wall, reflecting the back wards
of the familiar asylum.

Then resolve, the small spark of resilience.
Baby steps into the real, the helping hand grasped.

The pen, the instrument with which you navigate
the chaos, you journal and compose with. Progress evident
in the paragraph, the line. Complementary medicine
of the blackened page. A seasoned self emerges,
tempered in the flames of inspiration, the cool cast
of reflection. Recovery begins.

Dementia Praecox: early-onset dementia, the label used before "schizophrenia"
aphasia: inability to remember words; alogia: poverty of speech;
anhedonia: inability to feel joy;
anosognosia: loss of insight

SIDE EFFECTS

Dear Doctor: my vibrator is dressed in dust,
his batteries bleed acrid brown tears of loneliness and disuse.
The crochet club is appealing, something to keep
my once-nimble fingers in shape for the day
the old fire returns.

My lover has a choreographer and personal trainer
to bring these old bones to life; med-dead, I take hours
to ignite. Like a boy scout cursed with two green twigs,
he soldiers on against the odds of these damned antidepressants.

Sublimate, you say? I've no drive to deter.

Dear Doctor, my mind is quite steady,
but your potions have castrated me.
Humour me while I cackle in the dust
of my sensible underwear
at your question:

Are you glad
to be alive?

IMPERFECT PRESCRIPTIONS

"One pill makes you larger," the Jefferson Airplane sings, not meaning the obesity apparent in so many mental health clients, their slowed metabolism and increased appetites making them candidates for Type 2 diabetes.

Dry mouth, constipation, muscle stiffness, involuntary movements, especially of the mouth and tongue. Sexual dysfunction. Sedation. Agitation. Anxiety. The list of side effects is long and cruel.

At what cost sanity? A high price to be paid.

Imperfect prescriptions. Toxic remedy.
Chemical strait jackets.

IN THE SECOND PERSON

"And when you talk to yourself out of madness
it sounds at first like yourself, until you hit
upon the one word in your tired lexicon that
means "gentleness," and out of it comes the only
solution, *hope*, and out of supreme anger comes
compassion for yourself, the miracle, that there
are two in you, and one must pray to the other."
                    – Pier Giorgio Di Cicco, "Odes to the Just Society"

Schizophrenia: split mind. I spoke to myself in the second person
those days in the rooming house, when hallucinations played
hide and seek with my perceptions, and my nerves seared
on a hot wire wavelength. Moving photographs, statues mouthing
commands. Words writ large in indigo neon against
the whitewashed walls.

'You must,' I admonished
myself as I sat on the single cot in the small room,
thousands of miles from home.
'You should,' I advised
(pull myself up by my boot straps, face the music, stand steady
and all manner of clichés).

Higher self-conversing with the quotidian self.

Gentleness. I longed to bear its embrace.
But judgements rained down from my super ego,
that medicated and sane section of my mind. I would not let myself

off of the hook. I must toe the line. Where was God in all of this?

Absent.

Not for many years would I allow myself the luxury of prayer.

Recognizing hyper-religiosity as a symptom, I am able to navigate
the sacred inclination and still hold fast to lucidity.
Some would still say this is delusion.

The voice of angels is a whisper in an otherwise quiet mind.

IN DEVELOPING NATIONS

To haul water, to scrub metal pots with fine white sand,
to mind the elders, fetch their sweet tea and bathe their limbs,
to swaddle babes and rock their cradles – these are necessary,
and good acts, and I can do them, though my mind ignites
with a million phantoms jeering, their voices rattling
in my skull.

Second cousins, grandparents, siblings – all live within
shouting distance and know me from birth. I have a place
in this community, and they accept me for who I am.

This is why I fare so much better than my peers
in industrialized nations, with their improved health care,
welfare, asylums and mobile nuclear families.

Progress steals from the likes of me – the mad, who on
occasion lose touch with reality. My community tends to me
until I return, with tales from the other side, and perhaps
a holy vision or two.

INCANDESCENT (Brief Shining)

That there is no clearly defined "I" has caused
some maverick philosophers and anti-psychiatrists
to postulate those afflicted by schizophrenia
are closer to enlightenment than Normals.
Sifting delusion and word salads for truth,
hallucination for insight, these renegade scholars
wore their hearts on their sleeves, craved salvation,
synthesis. From the hell of psychosis to the heights
of omniscience, from paranoia to wisdom, prescience.

Better the syringe, the elixirs which broach schisms
between thought and affect, action. Better lucidity
than questionable prophecy, better a primer than
Nostradamus' cryptic stanzas. While only one sentence
in a monologue of years may come to fruition, I say
better the real, better the real.

BETTER THE REAL

No "I," but fragments, affect independent
of thought, action. Mad dog mind, hurling
itself at the perimeters of experience, chain
links of the perceived. From this, the cacophony
of tongues, perhaps prophecy a la Nostradamus,
something to be decoded. So said the renegades,
and gained favour for a season.

I say, "better the real!" the elixirs that tame
the rabid brain, right the chemistry, calm the body,

(Though I laid the Tarot, scried the crystal globe,
sat full lotus in clouds of sandalwood smoke,
seeking prescience.)

Better consensual reality than the slow burn
of a meteorite, illuminating the path ahead
before crashing: a cinder, a corpse.

BENZOS

This far from a cigarette, a drink,
a good hit of weed. Sober thoughts
don't always make sense. Pacing. Something
about loops. Obsession. I place the benzo
beneath my tongue, where it breaks down
into a sharp-tasting powder. PRN.
Highly addictive, but not at this dose,
I've been assured. It calms the tardive
dyskinesia of twitching eyes, loosens the cold
claws from the heart, slows and deepens
breathing. Panic: Hell for sure.

It's been a long time since menthol smoke
caressed my lungs with its cloud-coloured comfort,
sending energizing nicotine to my beleaguered
brain, assuaging the sedation. There's no doubt
a cigarette is good for the schizophrenic's thought
processes, but I'm done with that. I have my benzodiazepams.
PRNs. Emergency only. Those and my injections
of antipsychotics, and once-daily antidepressant tablets.
I'll survive the absence of cigarettes, the token
of the psych ward economy.

They say I'm clean and sober. But I am fueled
by chemistry. Leave it to the 12-Steppers
to determine.

DOWN THE ROAD

I went for a walk, legs moving through icy cold freedom,
the sidewalk clear of all but snow, stretching on into
the immediate future, a future without shackles or restraints,
not bordered by institutional walls.

And I breathed in, grateful.
And I sighed in relief.

I would not have to run, go on the lam, appear
before a tribunal. I was free, alive and living
in the community, indistinguishable from the mentally well,
by virtue of my treatment, with help from my reading,
programs, camaraderie. The support I received proved invaluable.
I could go for a stroll, unassisted, unchaperoned, in the wide
open spaces of my neighbourhood. I could choose
what to eat, when to retire, and whether or not I would
watch television. Or not.

I thought of peers in prison, the largest mental hospitals
on this continent, doing time for petty crimes
committed while delusional, left untreated, to languish
in solitary confinement, left to the mercy of other prisoners and
guards.

I recalled feeling imprisoned while in asylum, locked doors
and curfews, claustrophobic panic twisting my days.

I strode down the road, arms close by sides to hide the tremble,
resisting the urge to look over my shoulder.

TUITION FOR THE ASYLUM

Neurotransmitters, misfiring elixirs explode
in a shower of light. Molten tongues trace shivers,
music to seduce the blistering kiss.
Logic melts in the inferno.

Cabbalistic mystery of street signs.
Crucifixion plots of the office. Death's seduction,
the will to survive, wield razor-sharp symbols
in the arcane battle of wits.

Solitary cells of failed chemistry.
Haunted, inexorable faces. The incessant murmur
of monologues, awkward dances which signify occult
side effects.

Choreography of the present shift, the maestro
a cane-wielding dementia case.

If G-d is ancient, does he forget telephone numbers?
What is the future but a bend in the path?
Can't you see I'm busy saving the world
from linear delusion? Let me go!

TORTURED

A voice, believable as science, declares love
from the distance of lawns and fences.
Whose heart breaks here in this street
of constant construction? Or is it my mind,
hungry for such a shouted assertion?

I sit on the step, chain-smoking and lost
to reality's seduction. The birds scatter
over a cement spill, droppings like ill-fated
lovers' hearts, hardening in the new driveway.

The muscle of machinery flexes, muttered curses
and grunts amongst the roar and clang.

Easy to hear things when the birds are silenced,
I reason, take my cup inside, and hide
beneath the blackened sheets of scribblings,
cover my ears with my hands, pray for psychosis' retreat,
tortured into submission by a traitor brain.

THE WILL

Do not come knocking with your promises of nothing, your great
sleep, your ultimate solutions. I've tidied the rooms. I've taken
up with new causes. I've collected a pallet of potions to paint you
out of the picture. No, Suave Seducer, you are not welcome here.

I used to dance with you when words melted in required texts,
and your wheezy voice whispered in my mind's ear. I'd calculate
the leap from balcony to pavement, bridge to river. I'd plot
to procure the necessary chemistry, extinguish pilot lights, turn
up the gas. Ours was an intricate courtship.

After three dream-deprived nights I swallowed your bottle of courage,
chased by tequila. That cocktail was nullified by a soft swig of charcoal
the hospital barkeep proffered, and I was forced to live.

Now I peek behind curtains and around bends, fearful of your reap-
pearance. O, death, I've erected electric fences, wire taps and dug
moats. I've sealed myself off in a cloud of instinct. I've outgrown you.

POSTMODERN ASYLUM

Chrome and glowing glass, inlaid brick baroque
erased by rubber-soled nurses,
flowers dying in architectural arrangements
in gift shop refrigerators,
Third World crafts on fold-away tables.

In the corner, an art gallery, a small
solace of solitude to be savoured.

Sotto voce. Pre-med poseurs discuss ins and outs
in some lost language I'll never master
in this lifetime, while a transgender woman strokes
her hair, unaware the brow bone tattles
on the original gender.

The psychiatrist chases cures with a cell phone
glued to his ear, yay or nay a donkey's bray,
with Zarathustra taking dictation. We worship
where we should only observe.

Surreal landscape of the lower-floor maze
of mind doctors and the mad, cubicles
brimming with secrets, day passes burning
the palms of sweat-drenched, clenched fists.

In the penthouse of undulating pedways:
celestial skylights, long-term lunatics, babbles and moans,
hunger strikes and perversions, contraband commiserations.

Sandwiched between the freed and incarcerated insane –
cardiac cases, x-rays, ECGs, like quotes
in a text on mortality.

RECOVERY

"A home, a job, a date on the weekend" –
this is the experts' definition of recovery
from the most serious madness. This is
the gold standard the workers hold forth
when bending the will of the afflicted

To complete crafts, like papier maché,
or Sexton's moccasins, when guiding
the deluded through whittled-down daily routines.

I devour the literature on recovery like cheesecake,
taste buds singing for the tart flavour of hope
(so much work to be done).

I devote my limited energies to the task at hand,
remnants of my grandiosity whispering
in the corridors of my consciousness,
that my words, not the time cards of some factory,
will survive me.

I return to the pen when the dishes demand
washing, grateful no professional visits.

Guilty secret, this prioritizing for the future
while the present decays.

BEDLAM BECKONS

Bedlam beckons in the blear of night,
with its pretty packets of forget-me pills.
Its nurses, sparkling from afternoon naps,
padding softly with big-eyed lights.

The insomniac, veins like aqueducts,
fashions a shroud of bed sheets, shrieks
into the lead-heavy hours.

The corpse of compassion, secured to a gurney
by money belts and lawmen's holsters,
is destined for a return to the Middle Ages.

The residents, washed pale in disinfectant,
shuffle somberly or snore, tranquilized and vivisected
by the wave charting machine, cannot muster
the energy to stop their decay,

And, outside, the moon winks its orb
at the manicured lawn.

A HAVEN I HAVE KNOWN

I.

Wailing Johnny Cash blues into the yellow smoke
of the television room, grateful for the prepared meals
and monitored cell, the manse of the mind my home
for one solid month of defied orders
before I was discharged against better judgement
to flounder in the marketplace.

Phantoms danced across the ventricles of my broken
brain until I longed to return.

But there was no room, bulldozers ate through offices and wards.
Terrified patients fled the sinking ship to drown in the obscene
carnival of the streets.

II.

The bottle, the gutter, the grave
await the displaced; tranquilizer darts replace
art therapy, tattered robes on malnourished bones
decorate doorways and SRO holes.

Bleeding to feel more than dull defeat,
the disenfranchised confront the elite

Mere parasites to the cost-cutting crew,
less than human, less than well,
despite the concerted efforts of Big Pharma
and its many imperfect concoctions.

APPOINTMENT

I want to mould you
like clay, create a vessel
for my variations on the themes
of identity, autonomy
the enervating struggle for sustenance
of the mind and belly,
the nature of reality.

I want to fill your skull
with my words, let your vibrant brain
decipher the unconscious drives
bending my tongue and pen towards Babel.

I want you to pronounce me healed
with a flourish, in a ceremony of cymbals
and gongs, drums and rattles, the scents
of sandalwood and caribou hide filling the room.

But, alas, as I gaze over your shoulder
at the glaciers lapped by the sea,
I see an absence of footprints
on the waves, and resign myself
to your science and kindness
your imperfect prescriptions

The white noise and ionized air
of the hospital office

Where I check in at regular intervals.

SHRINKIPOO
(a study in transference)
(for Dr. G)

"Those who do not judge by appearances are shallow"
        – Oscar Wilde

I thought I would love you
for 56 days, my infinite compassion
a balm on your scars, the file on your desk
gently thickening into a poetic biography
suitable for publication. I offered myself
up for a cure, one you could make a name on,
but then you trimmed your moustache and hair,
rearranged your office, and began to look
like my uncle, so I returned the books
which offered all of the answers
and wrote you a prescription
for good chicken soup –

Another guru overthrown by circumstance.
And I, a would-be disciple, left chasing
my shadow in the autumn light of my 45th year.

CLINICAL OBSERVATION

I suspect my psychiatrist arrives at his office
while it is still dark, arms laden with garden blossoms,
leather-bound books, and limited-edition prints
rearranging the artefacts with care
each day at dawn
to save his own sanity
from the onslaught of woe.

There are reminders of his money,
red and gold, misty photographs of his summer view,
a few nostalgic texts from the 1970's
when he wore bellbottoms and had his hair long.

Lately he's displayed his knowledge of chemistry
and a jar full of dust, labelled "Ashes of Difficult Patients."

The latter makes me wince
and at turns vow to haunt him
in death as in life
with my suspicious nature, my demands.

He's grown a goatee and gotten a manicure.
The only thing missing is an ascot
and a pipe.

But he subscribes to *Runners' World*
and drinks citrus juice
in step with the times.

I survey the room
settle into the new furniture,
gaze at a spot to the left of his head
uncertain of where to begin.

I tick off new decorations
as I list my symptoms
driven to distraction by the desire to know
what he writes on the clean sheet of paper.

If it was me, I'd write a grocery list
a poem, or practice my signature,
bored by the usual refrain.

But the scenery keeps changing
and keeps him awake.

SEASONAL

Madness, come to call at Christmas,
remain until Valentine's, renders the world
small as a pearl and as pale. Odin winks
in greying drifts, sunlight rare and smudged.

> *(Please leave a message. I am nowhere*
> *to be found.)*

Love me/Love me not. Suicide notes bordered
by lace. Overdose with a wine's bouquet.
Humpty Dumpty has nothing on me, with my
hammering shoe, my self-help glue and welder's
torch of Reason.

> *Dear Doctor, dealer with degrees,*
> *the drugs you dole out, more pure than the harvest,*
> *explode like popcorn in the skull. Archaeologists*
> *of the mind, they unearth history, choreograph*
> *ghosts. They bring the sweet balm of sleep.*

> *You demand nothing but words, glimpses*
> *into the realms of lunacy, which you right*
> *with chemicals. Alchemist, you transform.*
> *Confidante, your lips are sealed as a tomb.*

Holy hosts beneath my tongue melt to calm.
I rest in the eye of a brainstorm, tra-la.

My shuffling gait. My stone face.

EDITOR'S NOTE

ky perraun's writing could be an excellent example of trying to heal feeling and thought even if they merge in uncertain ways. Cathartic distances with each poem's intimate dramas and her own recovery itself is something miraculous in establishing a personal distance from the 'sickness'. Like a curator, she places precise critical distances in the vast middle spaces between the sculpted image of perfect health and the Bosch-esque background of madness and its pale, wormy flesh in wild gardens.

Her ethical awareness shows the kind of empathy that has been lost at times, then found as an injured thing, a tear-porous, victim-symbol. Her text serves as a suggestion that more work can be done to examine the strange encounter with (pseudo and actual) science and madness. Madness, in the mind of perraun, with her intelligence and articulation, emerges with its own agenda to which she responds daringly.

At times an elegy against empirical absurdities, perraun's text depicts delusion that is self-conscious and yet contained, and uses the poem as an exactly right fit, not a verbal straight-jacket.

As the reader turns the pages, they sense a hidden narrative of incredible details and surreal excavations. This is a text often haunted by the past like a sadistically curious poltergeist rather than by a certain spirit. perraun recalls various treatments that attempted to wring the madness out of people, ranging from systematic drowning, being chained, violent incarceration, etc. It is a meditation and a record of how we would hope that there could be no more terrifying treatments than we have already seen and that a modest but possible progress could re-emerge in this historiographic archeology, even if that progress is debatable as she demonstrates.

The linguistic relationship with madness is a complex but rich one; the thoughts of madness, and their being written down, contain a reference to reality. perraun's work could be imagined as an act of will to stay in reality despite factors that would render this nearly impossible, and she is never permanently lost in a narrative herself. In a paradoxical dream allegory about insomnia, she is both guide and subject. As demonstrated by perraun's text, madness is intrinsically about suffering, even in its romanticization. perraun wills us to not forget that this is a lived reality of her own.

– Kristian Enright

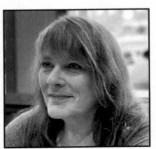

Photo: Izabela Ciechanowska

ky perraun is an Edmonton poet and writing group facilitator, who was diagnosed with schizophrenia in 1997. Having had her first poetry publication in 1983, while in journalism school, she continued submitting to magazines and anthologies throughout the decades, despite her diagnosis. In the early 2000s she helped form Right Heart Press, a micropress collective, which published her chapbook, *Paging Dr.G.*. In 2017 she received a Canada Council Cultivate Grant to produce a manuscript detailing schizophrenic treatments throughout history, which became *Miraculous Sickness*.